Why Weight? Change Now!

7 Secrets to Help You Lose Weight & Look Great!

Heather Farley

Published by
Brian Farley Ministries Incorporated, New York, New York

Unless otherwise indicated, all Scripture quotations are taken from the Holy Bible, New Living Translation, copyright © 1996, 2004, 2007 by Tyndale House Foundation. Used by permission of Tyndale House Publishers, Inc., Carol Stream, Illinois 60188.

ISBN: 978-1-7325917-0-7

TABLE OF CONTENTS

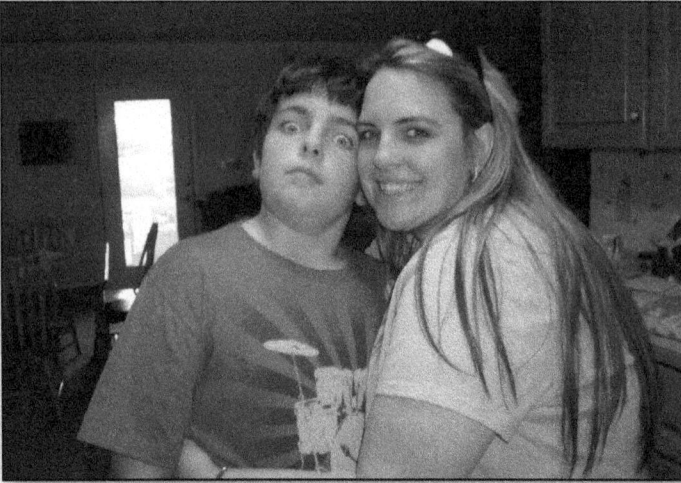

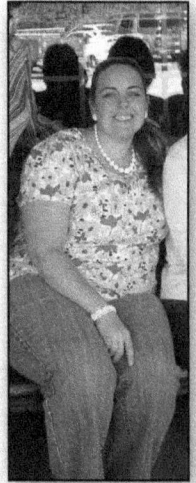

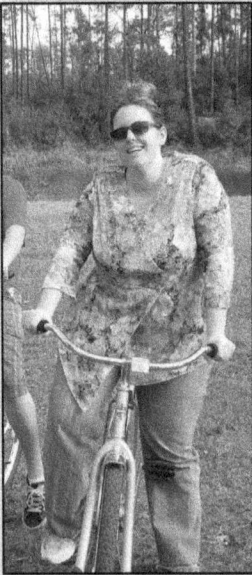

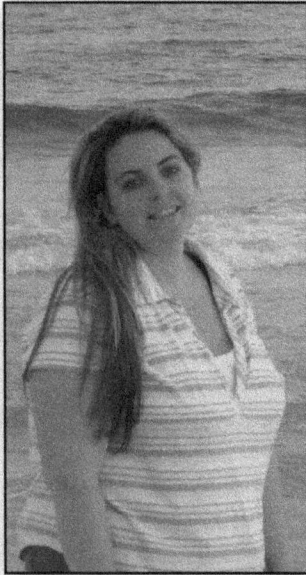

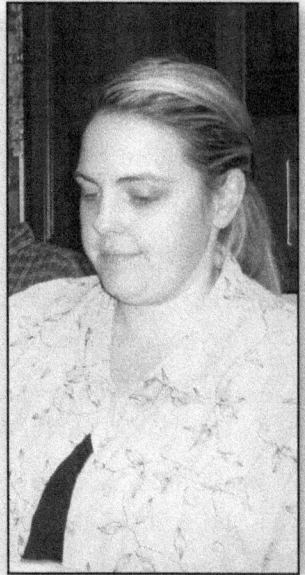

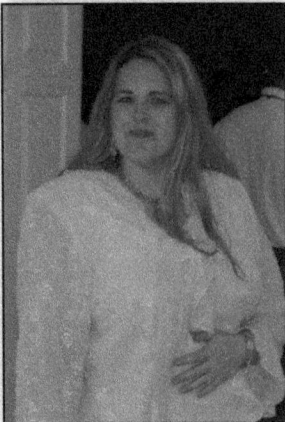

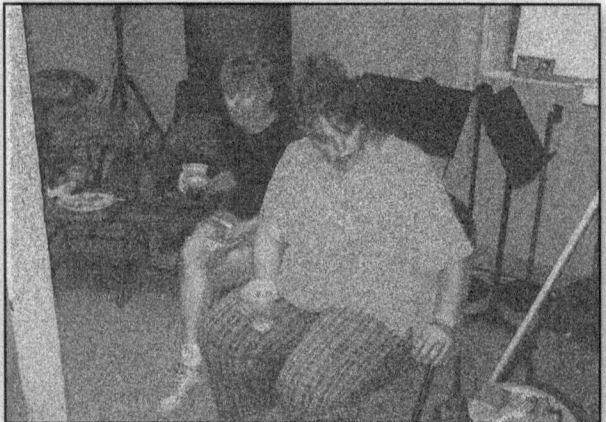

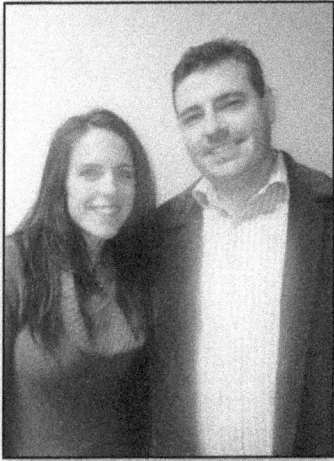
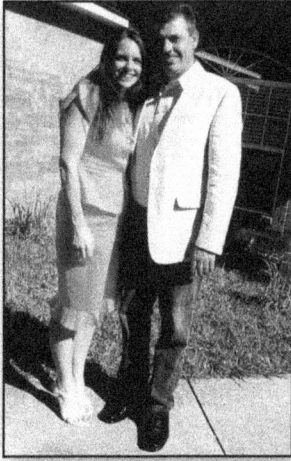
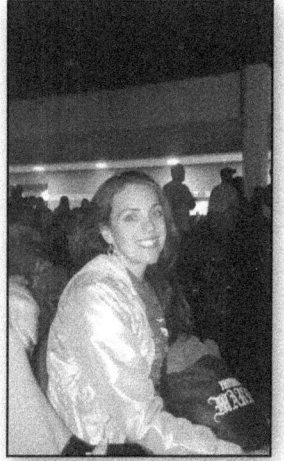
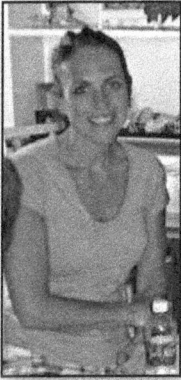
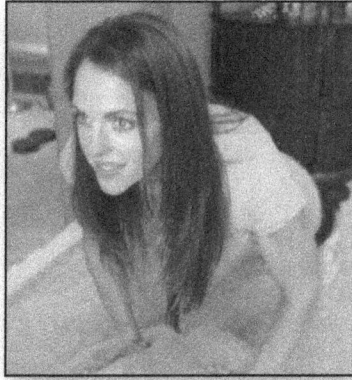
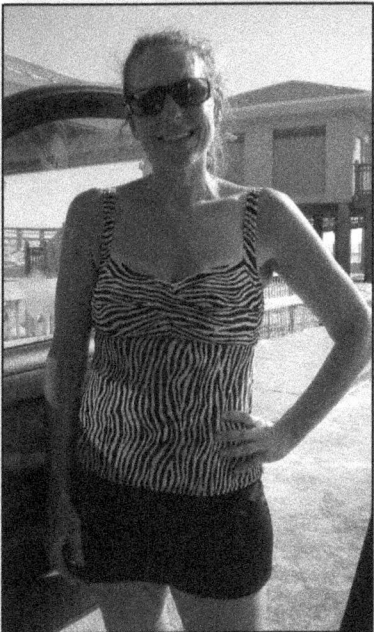
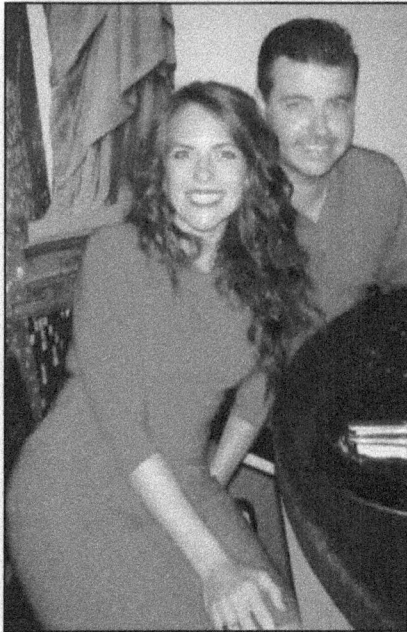

A LITTLE BIT ABOUT ME

I was born on October 11, 1974, and I weighed a little more than 7 pounds. I haven't always been overweight, but as far back as I can remember, I have been overweight! I believe my weight problem started when I was about 10 years old. I feel like I have tried every diet known to man and have been on a diet of some kind for most of my life. To name a few: I have tried the order your food by mail diets (lost about 25 pounds), store bought weight loss pills (lost 10 pounds), liquids only diet (lost a few pounds), Christian diet plans (lost 40 pounds), prescription diet pills (lost 20 pounds), more diet pills (gained 18 pounds back so started more pills - lost 11 pounds again), I have tried to eat only one meal a day, fasted for two days a week…all kinds of stuff. You name it, and I've probably tried it. It is possible that in all the diets together I may have actually lost more weight than I weighed at my heaviest!

My goal throughout most of my life was to be thin. Although I lost much weight with many of these plans, I was not changed on the inside, so I quickly gained the weight back…plus some more! If you have battled weight gain most of your life, then we have something in common. This is probably why you are reading this today. I am sure you have your own list of failed diet attempts and plans that resemble my list. Most likely, you are in search of answers, looking for the quick fix or the magic button to press in your mind to help you make the changes you need to make. The good news is I have an answer for you, the bad news is it isn't quick and it isn't painless, it isn't magic and it isn't easy.

Want some more good news? I see where the journey has been worth every mountain and trial. It has been worth every step that it took to climb. I don't regret ONE second of this journey. As a matter of fact, the journey to find myself has been more rewarding and fulfilling than I could have even imagined! But, since you don't know who I am let me tell you a little bit about me...

My name is Heather Farley. I am married to the world's most amazing, Godly man, Brian! We met at the age of 14. We lived on opposite sides of town (about 30 minutes apart). We went to different schools, but went to the same church. We actually disliked each other when we first met, but because the church was small with very few teens our age, it was hard to get away from each other! So we continued to hang out with the group. We found ourselves hanging out a little more, laughing about the same things, talking on the phone late into the night, driving across town to see one another. Before long, we were 'best friends'. That was what we had to tell our parents. You see, Brian was a bit of a 'player' when he was young, and his dad was tired of all the girls calling and leaving tearful messages on the answering machine for him to please call back. So he was restricted from having 'girlfriends'. Lucky for us, we had been friends for so long, we didn't even really know when the change from 'best friends' to 'boyfriend/girlfriend' happened. So they didn't either, (or at least they played along like they didn't for our benefit). In December of 1992, exactly 7 days before Christmas, we were married. It sounded sooo romantic at the time, however, we have discovered that is a really bad time to celebrate an anniversary. We usually try to celebrate in March or so, and the moral of this story? Get married in March! We have now been married more than 18 years. We had our first son, Aaron Joel in December of 1995 and our second son, Andrew Micah in July of 1999. Brian joined the United States Air Force shortly after we were married. We have been in pastoral ministry of some kind, part-time or full-time, for all of these years. After many years of moving around we moved back to Pensacola, FL in 2000 to plant a church in our home town.

We have been here ever since. God has done many amazing things, but that is a different story for a different day, although many of the events will play into the story I am sharing with you now.

Now you know a little bit about me, and who I am so let's get into why we are here.

The entirety of this book talks about what 'I' did to accomplish certain goals. I would like to begin the book by letting you know that the only way I reached any goal was by the help of the Lord Jesus Christ and His precious Holy Spirit. I could never have done anything without His help and guidance. So, as you read what 'I' have done, remember it is only Him working through me that I was able to accomplish these things. I give Him all the glory for that.

If you do not have a personal relationship with Jesus, and would like more information on how to begin a relationship with Him, please email me at pastorhfarley@gmail.com. All you have to do is accept that He is Lord. Jesus is Lord. That He was born of a virgin, that He died for your sins and made a way for you to be reconciled with the creator, Jehovah God. That He came back to life after being dead for three days. That He today is alive and well. He will one day return to take those who trust in Him to heaven with Him. You can ask Him to be your Savior and help you to find freedom. I promise, if you ask for His help, He will be proud to help you. He has been waiting your entire life for you to come to Him. He loves you!

WHY ARE WE HERE?

What has caused you to have any interest in reading this today? Are you overweight? Do you love someone who is? Are you looking for an answer, a way to lose weight once and for all? Are you tired of losing-gaining-losing-gaining? Well, if that is why you are here…..then you have come to the right place.

As I've already mentioned, I have tried many diets. I feel like I have been on a diet or weight loss plan all of my life! When I was a teenager and was dating my now husband I was a little smaller, but was still a 'plus size' about a size 16/18W. Then, through the years I continued to grow and shrink. Size 26W being my largest. My husband and I took a job as youth pastor at a church in Phoenix, AZ. Aaron was three years old and Andrew was four months old at the time of the move. Arizona is about a three day drive from Pensacola, FL, our home town, where all the grandparents and everyone who loved us lived. Needless to say I was extremely depressed while we were there. We were there only 9 months, but during that time I gained soo much weight. I remember getting on the scales one day and seeing a very scary number 265. I am only 5 foot 4 inches tall, so I decided at that point that something had to be done. I didn't have the emotional or physical strength to make it happen. So, I did what any good woman would do - I vowed to not step on those things again and to live in an imaginary world where I still weighed 220 pounds! Yes, still obese, but not 265 pounds! I did start walking some in the afternoons and at work on my breaks. I didn't really know where to start. I was overwhelmed, so large, out of control, and I just couldn't 'care' anymore. I felt it was hopeless to think that I would ever lose weight. Certainly NEVER even imagined that I might be an 'average' sized woman! That wasn't even allowed in my dreams. I was going to be satisfied with being a size 16/18W. If I could somehow just get back there I had decided I would be happy!

So the largest I have been was 265 (plus some). But 265 was the largest number I ever actually saw! I have read numerous books about 'eating disorders' and many of them put overeating and (bulimia/anorexia) in the same category. I am not judging those writers or their motives, but I question if they have ever had an eating disorder. I understand that they are saying that you have to 'love' yourself no matter what your size and how you got there. You see, I know in my heart and head that I should love myself at 265 pounds or 134 pounds, my weight shouldn't define my worth or who I am. But, knowing that and making it a reality, are two very different things. Well, that is just as simple as knowing in my head and heart that I should eat right and exercise everyday to be the person I want to be, but knowing it and believing it enough to act on it, to let it change who I am...well, those are two very different things!

I don't like to throw up, so I have NEVER understood wanting to eat a bunch then throw up (...oh wait...that's not true...there is one instance... but that story comes later) and anorexia? Really? If I was anorexic I wouldn't be fat, right? I'm sorry, but there is one thing that really gets on my nerves (well, there are many things, but one thing when considering weight and weight loss) the main thing that gets on my nerves is people who needed to lose 10 pounds trying to tell me how to lose weight. People, I weighed 265 pounds. I needed to lose 130 pounds or more. That is an entire person!! **If you have only lost 10 pounds, you couldn't help me!** Hey, I think losing 50 pounds is a great accomplishment, but even with that, you couldn't help me much. I needed to lose more than 10 pounds, I needed to lose more than 50 pounds, and I did it and so can you! The good news is if you only need to lose 10 pounds or 50 pounds, 150 pounds, or much more, the information I have will help you if you will let it. It will help empower you to change, so that those extra pounds will fall off. So, this book will focus mainly on being overweight and over eating. We will talk about how we use food for comfort, then find we are not comforted but just fatter, thus being more miserable, needing to eat more food to feel better and be comforted to just get fatter....It's a vicious cycle. I have lived this life and survived. I lost the weight and lived to tell about it! I went from a size 24 to a size 8 (I do even own a pair of pants that are a 6!) I now know, and believe it is possible for every person to do it as well. So here is my story. My prayer is that it will encourage you, inspire you and motivate you to change. You can leap into a new life of FREEDOM!

If it feels like a dream for you to find a healthy lifestyle, to lose weight, to change who you are, encourage yourself with this verse. Proverbs 13:19 NLT It is pleasant to see dreams come true, but fools refuse to turn from evil to attain them. **It IS possible to see those dreams come true.** Are you willing to turn from the evil parts in your life that have kept you there all these years? If so….your dreams can be attained! Trust me! If I did it, so can you!

I remember being a teenager and seeing talk shows where 'big' women would be talking about how they are 'happy' with their body. I remember thinking that was the place I needed to find. I needed to just find a way to be happy with my bigger body. I had been overweight my whole life, and was going to always be overweight. I should just figure out how to love myself in spite of the pounds. If you are overweight and happy then I think that is great. I am not doubting yours or these women's experiences, but I wasn't happy. I was miserable. I hated to go shopping, I hated to find clothes, I hated to go to big special events because I wanted to be 'cute' but felt that I wasn't. I have been a Christian since I was 16 years old. That has been more than 20 years. For 20 years I have been a Christian, wrapped in chains of fat, chains that held me captive. They were tight. I have been a worship leader for 10 years. Every time I got up in front of people I had to battle in my mind, "How can anyone even see God in me? I am a mess! People can see it every time they look at me." I allowed those chains to control my responses, not only in leading worship, but in every aspect of life and with everyone in my life. I know there were many opportunities that I didn't allow God to lead me through because I was so ashamed of who I was. This is one of the greatest tragedies of my life.

I knew if I was going to really change, I needed to discover where these chains were first wrapped around me. Through much prayer, self seeking and thought, I was given many answers. One of the first steps to breaking free from these chains that kept me in the cycle of using food for comfort was to discover when and why I started using it for that reason. Before we go any further, I realize there are many instances where people are overweight for medical reasons, and there may be nothing more they can do. But if you are reading this and immediately defending your weight we need to deal with that first thing. The reason that I know many of you are doing that is because I did it too! For years, I made excuses, defended my size and bad eating habits to myself. The most important thing you can do to change is to admit that you have a problem. You see, you can't fix or change something that you deny is even broken. One of the first steps to any program that works (like Alcoholics Anonymous) is to admit you have a problem.

So if you are saying,

1. "I do not use food for comfort!"
2. "Me and food have a very healthy relationship!"
3. "I exercise plenty, and I don't eat too many calories." Then, let me ask you a few questions....

Can I ask you to take this challenge? Write down what you have eaten for the last three days. How much you ate (calories) and when you ate. How much did you exercise in the last three days? How were you feeling when you ate that entire bag of powdered donuts? What was going on that day when you ate the whole bucket of ice cream?

I know for me a lot of my problem was eating too much fast food. I would go through a drive through all three meals everyday. I didn't want to spend the time and energy on eating right and cooking. The reason? I didn't care enough about myself to take the time to really care for me. When I began to add the calories of what all I ate everyday it is no wonder I didn't weigh 500 pounds or more! I was eating 1,000s of calories and well over 100 bad fat grams everyday. And exercise?? Are you kidding me? None! I didn't have 'time' for that. So, if you think maybe it is possible that just maybe you eat more than you should everyday, and just maybe you don't exercise enough, and just maybe you use food for comfort even just some times.....if maybe these things are possible, then let's move on. We will dig much deeper into these excuses and legitimate reasons for excuses in later chapters.

THE THREE DAY CHALLENGE

Day 1-

List of things I ate:

Food   Calories   How I felt

_____

_____

_____

Did I exercise today? How Much?_____

Day 2-

List of things I ate:

Food   Calories   How I felt

_____

_____

_____

Did I exercise today? How Much?_____

Day 3-

List of things I ate:

Food   Calories   How I felt

_____

_____

_____

Did I exercise today? How Much?_____

THE BEGINNING

Have you ever as an adult gone back to a place that you enjoyed or even hated as a child? For instance, a park that you went to many times as a child, or your elementary school, or an older church building? The rooms are so much smaller than you remember and the memories seem distorted because reality is so different from the memory you have.

The church I grew up in was a great place. When I was about 10 years old the church sold their current building to move to a newer, nicer location across town. We met in another building for a couple of years while the new church was being built. Many years later, as a young adult, I went back to that original building. I had all of these wonderful memories of the church building, things my friends and I would do and say, our secret hang outs, I remember the way the building looked and felt. Funny though, when I went back as an adult the building was very different than what I remembered. The paint was the same, the pews were the same, the stage and building layout didn't change, but the HUGE sanctuary that I would sometimes get nervous to sing in front of was not as huge (quite small actually) and the yard where we would run that seemed to go on for miles, was just a small lot of land. I said all that to say, "Our perceptions as children can sometimes be very distorted from true reality."

As children, because we are not adults and not yet mature, we see things very differently than how they really are. Before I dig any deeper into my story, I want to remind you that all of the experiences I faced were from my perception as a child; however, they were my perceptions, therefore they were real to me.

I wanted to tell you this for two reasons. The first reason is you need to understand that I love my parents very much. We have always had a good relationship. I KNEW that they loved me, even through the years of dysfunction we faced as a family. I would never even allow myself to deal with any 'bad' emotions that I was having because I thought them to be 'bad' or wrong or disrespectful. As an adult, I see where those perceptions and feelings that I had as a child should have been dealt with long ago. So, when you begin this chapter, I don't want you to do like I did for YEARS and keep yourself in this prison because you are afraid your feelings may be wrong or disrespectful. If they are what you perceived as truth, then they are real to you, and you need to deal with them for your own freedom. You will HAVE to deal with them to be free.

Secondly, I wanted to tell you that because I DID have a great family, I had a great support system. On most accounts my life was easy and great, and yet the enemy who comes to steal, kill and destroy somehow made it inside my peaceful little world. Through the years, I have read many books where women have had horrible lives. They tell these stories, stories that are horrific. I would think, "Well, my story wasn't like that, I must not have any emotional issues".

Your story doesn't have to sound horrific or devastating to have put chains around you. It just had to be real to you at the time. Satan can use anything to try and destroy you, even good things! In John 10:10 the Bible says, "The thief comes only to steal, kill and destroy." The enemy will use whatever he has. So, I want you to think hard. Dig deep. Consider where your bondage started. Do not just assume because you had a great life that you have no bondage.

I was blessed to be brought up in a Christian home. I was not abused in any way. I was very much loved and cared for by my family. I know that many people today cannot say that. Often women struggle with many issues because of events that happened in their childhood. I only had one issue to struggle with and to come to grips with. When I was in the sixth grade my parents divorced.

My mother, sister and I left our home that we grew up in and moved to an apartment just down the road. My father stayed in the house that we were raised in until he was able to sell it. Because my sister and I moved with my mother, we took most of the furniture out of the house. So, the house that I had known as my place of safety and rest was stripped of all of its comforts and was left basically desolate. To keep us going to the same schools and to be as safe as possible, I was left at this very empty, lonely, sad house for an hour or so every morning and a couple of hours in the afternoon. I was able to walk to and from school from the original 'family' home. This was the best plan at the time.

I wasn't allowed to go outside to play after school because that wasn't safe. You see my parents loved me and did an awesome job of protecting me, so I was trapped in this tomb of a house every day. Trapped to remember what was, trapped with my thoughts of trying to discover ways that I could have made things better, ways I could have changed to help my family stay together. I was desperate to stop these bombarding thoughts, so I would turn on the television and watch Brady Bunch reruns and eat... and eat....and eat. That was the only thing that would take my mind off of what was happening around me. Oh, how it brought me comfort and pleasure and what a distraction food became.

We didn't have much money and after the divorce, money was even more scarce for a while. So I would 'experiment' with different things in the kitchen, strange and different things that I could eat. I know on more than one occasion if there was nothing sweet in the house I would take a slab of butter and stir in some sugar. At the time, that was a pretty tasty dessert. (YUCK!) My chains were first locked on, at that moment, and from that time forward, the chains were just added, event after event, problem after problem, year after year, until they had gotten so long and thick that I was miserable and could no longer hold myself up. That was the place I found myself three years ago. And that was where my freedom process began.

You see for years I had used food not only as a means to fill my time when I was bored but it became a way to comfort myself and distract myself from the heartache and trouble around me. Many people turn to other things: alcoholism, drug addiction, sexual addiction, excessive spending, etc. But, my vice of choice was food. As if using food for entertainment wasn't enough, I also used it for comfort. I literally stuffed my emotions down with cupcakes and chips or anything else I could find. The night that my mother took my sister and I out of the home we grew up in I was told, "Heather, your sister looks up to you. She will be very upset with this news. We need you to put on a smile and act happy. Act like it is going to be a lot of fun. Tell her the good things. You will get two Christmas celebrations and birthday celebrations." My parents telling me that just added more chains. Again, that wasn't their intention. They were doing the best they could with a bad situation.

Rather than be sad about this life changing event, the fact that I felt like they were ripping the rug right out from underneath me, despite the fact that my life and world as I knew it was 'no more', I perceived that my job was to put on a smile and 'fake' happiness for the sake of my sister. I am a people pleaser by nature. That is what I like to do. I want people in my life to be happy and I want them to be happy because I help them be that way. I have no idea if this behavior started on this day or if I was born that way, but I knew I had to do what I was instructed, and I gave the best performance of my life. I slapped on my smile and sold it the very best I could to my younger sibling. Not knowing the consequences that would follow me from that day forward.

Again, I don't hold my parents responsible for this. I have forgiven them of any fault I had originally blamed on them. I have a wonderful, close relationship with both my mother and father. I did go through a time in my life that I resented them and their choices of course, doesn't every teenager/young adult go through this phase? Where you think your parents are to blame for all of your life 'issues' and problems? You really believe it is their fault and I guess to some degree it is partially. But remember, I told you, for the most part, I had good, Godly, Christian parents that loved me. They just had a time in life where they went a little 'crazy', but I know they did the best they could at the time. As an adult now having my own children to reckon with, and the perspective of a pastor's wife of many hurting people, it makes it much easier to see that life can slap you around and cause you to do things you never thought you would. It certainly takes away a judgmental attitude. So, it is not their fault that I have this issue, it is just the battle I was called to war. It is the cross I was called to bear. It is the adventure I was called to run through. However, I can now see where I allowed this event to set a very destructive pattern in my life to follow. I realized that I could slap on that grin and make everything seem good and happy, and never shed a tear, but there had to be some way for me to be comforted and the way I chose that comfort was in a nice plate of food. A box of pizza perhaps, a bag of chips, an ice cream bar or two, or five. Food and I had become so well acquainted, and I knew the comfort it possessed, that it was easy to rely on it for more than nutrition.

Of course, God turns the bad things in our lives into very good things. In the Bible, Romans 8:28 says," And we know that in all things God works for the good of those who love him, who have been called according to his purpose." Through a long series of events, I met my husband because of the divorce. Chances are I would not have met him if my parents stayed married and continued attending the same church. Brian is the greatest blessing of my life, so I am very thankful.

You can clearly see, diets in and of themselves were never going to help me. Sure, when things were going well and life was tolerable, I could stick to any crazy diet, but as soon as an event happened or a stressful time came, I immediately ran back to food. I used to tell people, "I can't lose weight because I LOVE food! There is hardly anything I don't like to eat". It was easy to find comfort in it, such a wide variety!!

I was in chains and I had to break free!! So I began to pray and fast. I wanted the Lord to know I was serious! I wanted freedom, and I had no idea how to be free. I wanted Him to show me. I was willing to give up 'good tasting' (actually very unhealthy) foods so He would talk to me and tell me what to do. I wasn't playing, I really meant business.

So my next question for you--are you serious? Do you mean business? Are you serious? **Are you really ready to change?**

Those closest to me, who saw the transformation ask me all the time, "What did you do? Tell me what you ate, how you exercised, EVERYTHING you did in detail" So here it is! This plan may not work for everyone, but this is what worked for me. You can take parts and pieces and make up your own plan with some of the information I provide if this plan will not work for you. I'm going to give you some "magic tricks" that worked for me, hopefully they will work for you too! Well, they are not actually "magic" they are learned disciplines that require self denial and total reliance on the Holy Spirit.

CHAPTER THOUGHTS:

MAGIC TRICK NUMBER 1

Prayer and Fasting

So I turned to the Lord God and pleaded with him in **prayer** and petition, in **fasting**, and in sackcloth and ashes. Daniel 9:3 NIV

Let me reiterate here, **you must be ready for a change**. You must be desperate to make a change, to really change. The definition of the word change according to Mirriam Webster is: to make different in some particular, to make radically different, to give a different position, course or direction to, to undergo a modification. You must be willing to do whatever you have to do to change. To actually modify who you are! If you have tried other diets and failed, if you have succeeded at times and failed later-you have just been dieting. What I am telling you is NOT about a diet. It is about changing who you are! From the inside out! I couldn't stand myself any longer and knew that something had to be done. I did the only thing I felt that I knew was left, the last resort. Isn't it funny how we go to the ONE who knows all the answers as a last resort?

I went to my Creator and asked Him for help! I prayed more than once for Jesus to show me what I needed to do to change. He has all the answers, and that should be the first place that we turn, but often it is not. And when we FINALLY decide to ask Him for help, He is waiting so eager to assist us because He loves us - really loves us! He wants what is best for us and has all of the answers we need. We will not find them anywhere else so really, turning to Him is the best thing you can do. So, I prayed and told Him that I was really, really ready and would do whatever He said to do. Here's what happened next....

Every year our church does a church wide Daniel Fast from January 1st-21st. A Daniel Fast comes from eating as Daniel ate rather than eating as the other king's servants did in the book of Daniel chapter 1 in the Bible. Let me give you a brief summary of that story. Daniel was a captive and was taken to live with the king. He was being trained by the king to be in his royal service. The king only selected the strongest and smartest to work for him. They were to be trained for three years. The king offered all kinds of foods and wine to the men in training, but Daniel asked that he not eat it, and instead eat only vegetables, fruits and natural foods with water. After a time, the king's staff saw that Daniel and his friends were the healthiest of all, so they allowed them to continue this diet during their training. In Daniel chapter 10, we see where the answers to his fasting and choosing to eat the right foods paid off. We see a conversation between himself and an angel that is important. We see where God protected him and gave him many answers. The ability to interpret dreams and gave him favor with the king. So when we fast we are doing a few things. The main thing being, we are making a sacrifice. We are saying that hearing the voice of the Lord in a particular situation is more important to us than eating food. In the case of a Daniel Fast we are saying that we will eat only healthy foods to purify our bodies and at the same time ask the Lord to speak to us concerning His plans and goals for our lives.

As we began the Daniel Fast in January 2008, for 21 days I ate fresh fruit and veggies. I was so strict that I lost about 18 pounds during those 21 days and had a great time doing it. I heard so much from the Lord during that time because I was crucifying my flesh for those 21 days and praying a lot.

I told the Lord that getting to know Him, and hearing from Him was more important than eating food. It was a fun time to be so close to Him. Of course, on day 22 I was ready for a pizza, a cheeseburger, a slice of cheesecake and a super sized Dr. Pepper. I immediately went back to my old eating habits. Then, in June we did another summer Daniel Fast. At that time, I decided I would never have Dr. Pepper again and only have diet drinks. I thought, "This is so crazy. If I can go for 21 days without this I can go forever." So I got rid of regular Dr. Pepper forever. I stuck with that with no problem and was happy with the change. I knew when I did that, it was easy, and I was ready for more, so much more. I had failed so many times and was so scared to even THINK about changing that I wasn't sure where to begin. I already was thinking about when I would 'quit dieting' (fasting) and eat something good again. Beginning in October, I knew I really wanted to change and began to seek the Lord and ask Him, "What exactly do I need to do to change, to really change. Not just diet, but change my life?" I saw an article in a magazine I was reading advertising the book, "Never Say Diet" by Chantelle Hobbs. The Holy Spirit spoke to me, "Start there, read that book. It will show you where to begin." I bought the book, but I kept it in a box through Thanksgiving and Christmas. I wanted to enjoy my last and final meals and parties with no thought of that book and what I was going to have to give up. (Because at that time I still thought I was just giving up something that I loved for a time. I had no idea what the Lord had in store for me when I bought that book.) Fasting is a powerful tool! Read the story of Esther from the Bible. An entire nation was saved because of fasting. Don't underestimate the power or fasting.

At the end of December, I pulled that book out and read what I was going to need for this new 'diet.' January 1, 2009, I started the Daniel Fast again. The previous year I had made a new friend. She and I went to a ladies retreat together, went to lunch several times and began talking a lot together. I learned from our conversations that because of medical issues she had, she chose not to eat a lot of things, things that she would actually like to eat. She had no weight struggle, but had to give things up for her health. When she would tell me these stories I would think, "she is so disciplined to be able to say 'no' to these things, I need to do that too because the way I am eating is making me miserable. If she can do it so can I!" So, I asked the Lord to help me do this. As I started it the Lord began to show me how to break free from my chains. The first thing He asked me to do was to "stay on the Daniel fast until further notice." He wanted to teach me several things through this.

The first thing He taught me was self control and discipline. I only ate Daniel fast approved foods. (a list of foods will be included at the end of the book). **He showed me that I DO have the power within me, through HIS Spirit, to overcome and have self control over food or any addiction.** That I COULD control the food that entered my body and it didn't have to have control over me any longer.

He showed me that I could survive on these foods, they were the best foods available and I would be fine. Eating healthy is expensive and I had to determine that I wasn't going to worry with cost. **Everything in life worth doing has a cost.** I would give up other things if I had to, but eating healthy was becoming a priority. I was committed to do what needed to be done to change. I no longer thought about cost. I bought what I needed to survive. I just ate fruits, vegetables, nuts, brown rice and beans...for days...for weeks...for months! The Lord was teaching me self control and I was proud of myself because I was learning it. He wanted to show me that I had to control my horrible habits of food addiction. I didn't eat meat, dairy, sugar or bread (anything you may consider delicious) until May. Even then, I was reading that I needed more protein for weight training and building muscle, so I decided to add protein to my diet by adding low fat dairy: cottage cheese, yogurt, fat free some cheese and eggs. I didn't add meat of any kind until June. The most important thing He taught me was reliance on Him. He showed me that I couldn't make it on my own. That I needed His help and strength to be successful. He showed me I have the power within me, through Him, to accomplish much more than I thought was possible. And finally, He taught me I could trust Him. You see, I had been a pastor for many years, helping other people with their problems and issues but I never really dealt with my own. When I asked my Creator to make me new and change my thinking, He was ready and willing.

Why did I run to food? Well, we all run to something when we are hurting. Our past experiences often dictate what we run to until we make the choice to change. We must run to Jesus. He is the only one who can bind our wounds, heal our hearts and lead us out of bondage into freedom.

Everywhere we turn to except Christ is a dead end!

There is a pretty big factor that needs to be included here. Which leads me to Magic Trick Number 2.

CHAPTER THOUGHTS:

I will begin a fast on _____.

I will fast from_____.

I will pray at_every day for minutes._____

DANIEL FAST FOODS

Foods you may eat:
- Whole grains:
- Brown rice, oats, barley
- Legumes:
- Dried beans, pinto beans, split peas, lentils, black eyed peas
- Fruits:
  Apples, apricots, bananas, blackberries, blueberries, boysenberries, cantaloupe, cherries, cranberries, figs, grapefruit, grapes, guava, honeydew melon, kiwi, lemons, limes, mangoes, nectarines, papayas, peaches, pears, pineapples, plums, prunes, raisins, raspberries, strawberries, tangelos, tangerines, watermelon
- Vegetables:
  Artichokes, asparagus, beets, broccoli, Brussels sprouts, cabbage, carrots, cauliflower, celery, chili peppers, corn, cucumbers, eggplant, garlic, gingerroot, kale, leeks, lettuce, mushrooms, mustard greens, okra, onions, parsley, potatoes, radishes, rutabagas, scallions, spinach, sprouts, squashes, sweet potatoes, tomatoes, turnips, watercress, yams, zucchini; veggie burgers are an option if you not allergic to soy.
- Liquids:
  Spring water, distilled water, 100% all-natural fruit juices, 100% all natural vegetable juices.
- Others:
  Seeds, nuts, sprouts

Foods to Avoid:
- Meat
- White rice
- Fried foods
- Caffeine
- Carbonated beverages
- Foods containing preservatives or additives
- Refined sugar
- Sugar substitutes
- White Flour and all products using flour
- **Margarine, shortening, high fat products**

Fasting Resources: *http://www.billbright.com/howtofast/ http://www.worldprayercenter.org/beta/images/PDF/2007%20magazine.pdf http://www.inplainsite.org/html/fasting.html http://www.allaboutprayer.org/ prayer-and-fasting.htm http://www.new-life.net/fasting.htm http://www. freedomyou.com/level%202/Fasting%20Page%20G uide.htm*

MAGIC TRICK NUMBER 2

-Obedience

The Bible says in James 1:25, But if you look carefully into the perfect law that sets you free, and if you do what it says and don't forget what you heard, then God will bless you for doing it.

We took our churches' youth to a conference in January 2009. The 'theme' of the conference was freedom. The speaker for the conference was Eddie James. The thought and plan for the teens was freedom from sexual sin, freedom from drug addictions, freedom from alcoholism: many things young people struggle with today. The funny thing is, freedom is freedom! The Lord used this youth conference to minister freedom to me. As the leader of the worship service was talking, the Lord said to me, "If you will obey me, I'll show you how to lose weight. If you will obey, I'll teach you how to do it and make it happen, but you have to be willing to obey me." Remember, I had been fasting and this trip came on day 22 of the fast, but God had asked me to keep going with the fast, and I was thrilled to do so because I loved the closeness that I felt while fasting.

Well, you will never guess what He told me to do next. You will never guess what set of instructions He asked me to follow next. He asked me to, "Get out in the aisle and dance. Dance like you are free! Dance as if you were free from being unhealthy and overweight!" Well, I was standing in the back of this auditorium with thousands of teens. Many of them were dancing, jumping and singing for their own freedom. They were not even interested in what I was doing. I was just some 'old woman' to them. However, there is something about doing all the dancing and jumping yourself. I thought for a minute, "Lord! You know I can't dance! I can sing, but dancing has never been something I am good at! Lord, there are teenagers all around! They don't want this big woman dancing, they just want me to sit quietly in my chair!"

The Lord had just given me seemingly easy instructions, asking me to obey Him, then giving me clear direction towards the first steps. The next move was mine to make. Many of you, if you would be willing to open your heart to the voice of the Lord, He would speak to you. He would give YOU instructions and He would guide you. The question is would you obey Him when He did? You see, I didn't have to dance that night to lose weight. I had to dance that night to show God I was serious and to prove to myself that I would in fact obey what He told me to do. If I couldn't do THAT tiny little thing, there was no way I would be able to do the things He would be asking of me later! So, I stood there for a minute, deciding if it was what I REALLY wanted. Deciding if freedom was worth this price I was being asked to pay. I decided it was. I scooted past my husband and got into the middle of the aisle. I did a little 'foot movement'. You see, for all of the people around me, this was nothing. They didn't care what I was doing. It was a powerful service. Many people were being delivered from their own struggles and battles.

I would dare say that the people who knew me on the trip had no idea what was happening at that moment and what a momentous, miraculous moment it was in my life. We often allow Satan to hold us back with his lies, and his lies keep us in chains. I have told several in the group that year this story. They don't even remember me being out there dancing. They hardly even remember that trip. That has been years ago, and to teenagers, that is a life time! So don't let the devil lie to you and keep you bound. Be willing **Obedience is doing what I know I should do, even when I don't feel like it!** I still struggle with making these choices! If I want to lose weight and get healthy then I have to control how many calories I am taking in each day. If I want to be healthy I have to exercise. There are days that I don't WANT to do those things. I WANT to just eat and eat for comfort, and I WANT to stay in my house and not move. There are many mornings I WANT to hit snooze and just sleep through my run. But, if I'm going to obey what the Lord has told me, then sometimes I have to do what I don't feel like doing!

The Lord gives us many scripture promises to stand on and believe in. His Word IS the perfect law and it will set you free if you will allow it to. If you do what it says and don't forget what it says, God will bless you! One of my favorite scriptures that I have come to love is from Psalm 119:73 (NLT) You made me, You created me. Now, give me the sense to follow Your commands!" The Lord will do that for you! If you will ask Him and trust Him and obey Him - He will give you the sense to do what His Word says! He will give you the power and knowledge to be free! The Lord loves you! **The One who created you has a desire to make you all that He intended for you to be.** He is willing to give you instruction and guidance. You must be willing to receive His words and be willing to make the changes! If you have given your life to Jesus Christ, you have the power inside of you to be free! You have the power inside of you to say NO to the desires that have kept you in chains for a lifetime! to obey the Spirit of God! Be free in Jesus NAME!

CHAPTER THOUGHTS:

For many God will not ask you to get in the aisle and dance (He may). What He does tell you to do, will you do it?

What is the Lord speaking to me to change? What things can I do to obey Him?

MAGIC TRICK NUMBER 3

-Forgiveness

Look at this story from Matthew 18:21-35 NLT[21] Then Peter came to him and asked, "Lord, how often should I forgive someone who sins against me? Seven times?"[22] "No, not seven times," Jesus replied, "but seventy times seven,[23] "Therefore, the Kingdom of Heaven can be compared to a king who decided to bring his accounts up to date with servants who had borrowed money from him. [24] In the process, one of his debtors was brought in who owed him millions of dollars. [25] He couldn't pay, so his master ordered that he be sold—along with his wife, his children, and everything he owned—to pay the debt. [26] "But the man fell down before his master and begged him, 'Please, be patient with me, and I will pay it all.' [27] Then his master was filled with pity for him, and he released him and forgave his debt. [28] "But when the man left the king, he went to a fellow servant who owed him a few thousand dollars. He grabbed him by the throat and demanded instant payment. [29] "His fellow servant fell down before him and begged for a little more time. 'Be patient with me, and I will pay it,' he pleaded. [30] But his creditor wouldn't wait. He had the man arrested and put in prison until the debt could be paid in full. [31] "When some of the other servants saw this, they were very upset. They went to the king and told him everything that had happened. [32] Then the king called in the man he had forgiven and said, 'You evil servant! I forgave you that tremendous debt because you pleaded with me.[33] Shouldn't you have mercy on your fellow servant, just as I had mercy on you?'[34] Then the angry king sent the man to prison to be tortured until he had paid his entire debt.

[35]"That's what my heavenly Father will do to you if you refuse to forgive your brothers and sisters[e] from **your heart."**

You must be willing to forgive.

My whole life, I THOUGHT, I had forgiven my parents. I thought I was over it, but when I started praying and really thinking about where this food prison really began He revealed so much to me. I realized that I had chosen to suppress those feelings of resentment. That I had chosen to not really deal with them at all. I thought, and felt like, these emotions were 'wrong' and 'bad' or somehow disrespectful therefore I would not even allow myself to think about them. For all these years, I was carrying around this burden of un-forgiveness, and it had me locked in a prison! So I prayed this simple prayer,

"Lord, I know that my parents did not hurt me on purpose. I know that they were just entangled in sin, as we all are for a season, and that they loved me. **I know that at any moment those same choices they made could be made by me.** They didn't intend to hurt me. Just as Jesus prayed to You as He hung on the cross, "Father forgive them for they know not what they are doing" I pray that. And I declare that. I know they had no idea what consequence this would cause for me, and I choose to forgive them and release them of any fault that I have placed on them for their actions."

I know it was my choice to over eat and not exercise, but I had to forgive them for the hurt that I felt.

I have to tell you, I didn't feel the earth shake or hear thunder when I prayed this, but I believe there was a supernatural release of the prison chains as I chose to forgive them. I don't only believe it, I know it. According to the scripture that you read, if we choose not to forgive we will be sent to prison and tortured. Now, the Bible presents this as a literal prison with bars and guards and such.

I believe that it was a story to show us the same is true today. When we choose to hold onto un-forgiveness, we are put in a prison in our minds. We are tortured by our past hurts, and we cannot break free from unhealthy habits and life cycles that we find ourselves in because that bitterness and un-forgiveness keeps us chained up.

I was ready to be released, are you? If so, take the time now to stop and think about where your prison really began. Release forgiveness for the sins you perceive were committed against you. Release that burden and see your prison cell open!

Once you forgive, move out of the past and into the future. Focus on the days ahead!

That is why we never give up. Though our bodies are dying, our spirits are being renewed every day. [17] For our present troubles are small and won't last very long. Yet they produce for us a glory that vastly outweighs them and will last forever! [18] So we don't look at the troubles we can see now; rather, we fix our gaze on things that cannot be seen. For the things we see now will soon be gone, but the things we cannot see will last forever. 2 Corinthians 4:16-18

You may have one of those horrific stories that I spoke of earlier. Maybe your story isn't as 'easy' as mine. Whatever caused your chains, whatever keeps you bound up, let it go. Forgive and move on. It is the only way to be truly free! Don't dwell on the past or even the present. Look to the future. Look to what Christ has for you, your reward.

12 I don't mean to say that I have already achieved these things or that I have already reached perfection. But I press on to possess that perfection for which Christ Jesus first possessed me. 13 No, dear brothers and sisters, I have not achieved it, but I focus on this one thing: Forgetting the past and looking forward to what lies ahead, 14 I press on to reach the end of the race and receive the heavenly prize for which God, through Christ Jesus, is calling us.

Philippians 3:12-14

CHAPTER THOUGHTS:

1. Identify the people and the circumstances that played a role in the battle of your addiction.
2. Identify your role in choosing to sin in these areas.
3. Meditate on scripture about forgiveness.
4. Pray. Pray out loud or write your prayer in a journal. If you are having a hard time coming up with a prayer then use mine from earlier in the chapter, just insert your circumstances and story in the blanks.

Who do I need to forgive?

What are some things I can think about that were painful and I know I need healing from?

Ask God right now to begin healing those places, cry, mourn, live those moments and let God heal your heart.

I chose to forgive for_____.

"Lord, I know that __did not hurt me on purpose. They were overtaken by their own ability to sin. I know that at any moment those same choices they made could be made by me. Just as Jesus prayed to You as He hung on the cross, "Father forgive them for they know not what they are doing" I pray that. And I declare that. I choose to forgive them and release them of any fault that I have placed on them for their actions."

MAGIC TRICK NUMBER 4

-Don't Be Afraid Of The Transformation!

Do not conform any longer to the pattern of this world, but be transformed by the renewing of your mind. Romans 12:2a
For the first five months of this adventure I ate very healthy. I wrote down EVERYTHING including the calories, fat, protein, fiber content of each item that I consumed. EVERYTHING! I had to have accountability. I know better than to trust myself because I LOVE food, and I have a tendency to want to cheat!

Also, while I was learning about self control, I had to be controlled. With no cheating! I had the support of my wonderful husband and children. They have lived with me through many diets, many attempts and I appreciate them not taking this opportunity to remind me of all the times I had tried and failed, rather they went along with all of my requests. My husband had a hard time with this because he loved me all along and didn't understand why I did not love myself as much as he loved me. But he respected my decision to try and make the changes. The first thing was I didn't cook for them. Now, some of you may be saying, "I can't 'not' cook for my family." If this is a big deal to your husband and your children then by all means keep peace in your home, but there are many things you can do.

For example, there were many church events where we would have people over. If I was cooking a meal for others I would be sure and have something delicious available for me to eat. A bowl of grapes to chew on or a bowl of carrots, while I prepared. I would eat a snack or a meal before I prepared and served food for the others, that way I wasn't as hungry, so it wasn't as tempting. If you have to cook for your family, then you have to, but for me, I couldn't or I would eat it. I had to resist temptation of any kind to build up my faith and build my self control.

I asked my three 'boys' if they were going to eat out (which they did often) to please not bring it in the house. I laughed one day when they all came home; and I heard them pull in the driveway, but I knew it was several minutes before they came in the house. I asked them when they came in where they had been. My sons looked a little upset because they were instructed not to tell me where they had been. Finally one of them spilled the beans, 'We went through the drive through but knew you didn't want it in the house. So daddy made us eat outside then throw the trash in the can outside, so you wouldn't have to see it or smell it".

Of course I laughed and that was a proud moment for me. Some of you may be reading this and thinking that is taking it to the extreme. Maybe so, but I am good at sneaking a fry here or there, a bite of this burger and that. I had to take DRASTIC measures to really change, so they were on their own with meals. I did provide them with things they could make on their own; sandwiches, mac and cheese, frozen dinners, etc, but I didn't cook big 'delicious' meals for many months or eat out with them at all. We eat out more than most because we are pastors, and it seems that much of our job revolves around eating with people. For the first year (which was my strictest training season) I chose to have people over to the house for meals rather than make plans to eat out. That way I could better control the menu choices and the calories I would be consuming.

This point is a pretty big one. Probably the biggest in the whole message I am sharing here. **You HAVE to be willing to change your life.** (have you heard this yet?) You HAVE to be willing to give up some stuff that you may love to gain the better things in life. You must be willing to make temporary sacrifices to gain permanent change. As pastors we see people all the time addicted to drugs and alcohol. Some of these people often have opportunities to go to rehabilitation centers to get help, but they make excuses as to why they can't go, "I can't not work for that long" or "I can't leave my family." Yes, it would be hard on them. Yes, it would be a sacrifice for a while, but the real answer they are giving is just a big fat "No!" to the changes that need to be made. In times past my husband has pulled strings to get men into treatment facilities, but the first time some are confronted with their sin, they begin to blame others and leave. They just aren't willing to change. The same is true for weight loss. You have to be willing to change your life. You can't keep living your life the same way you have lived it at 100, 200 or more pounds overweight and just think that because you want to now change that things are going to change automatically. No, you have to make actual changes and plan for success.

I had to get all snacks out of my house. I had to NOT buy groceries that would tempt me. I had to tell my kids and husband, "this is really important to me. I do not like the way I look and feel anymore, and I want to change it. It is going to take some time and for now you are on your own for feeding unless you want to eat what I am eating" (which they did not at the time, but they have all made major changes just from my changes!)

While we are on this thought of making changes, let's go ahead and discuss the dreaded word you have been waiting to hear…..yes, exercise. Exercise is a central key to healthy weight loss. Your body needs you to move! I can tell you every time I have missed exercise over the last two years and it hasn't been often. If you are reading this and ready to quit because you hate that word and the thought of exercise, let me tell you, you are in good company. I hated getting hot. I hated getting sweaty. I hated moving. In the summer I didn't want to be hot, and in the winter I didn't want to be cold. I could come up with an excuse to not exercise any day of the week. My life was and still is BUSY! My husband and I pastor a church. I have two children running in opposite directions.

There was and still is, always someone needing my time and attention. These were ALL good excuses and legitimate reasons to NOT exercise. The problem with all of the excuses, is they were not going to make me healthy and they were not going to help me lose weight. I had to be willing to, and here is this word again, be willing to CHANGE! You have to be willing to change. I had to give up many things to make this new lifestyle change! In February 2009, a friend paid the first month's fee for me to join a health club, 123 Fit. It was a small, little place with not many people. I liked it there because I didn't have to see many people. I would go in for 30 minutes a day and work out. I rode a bike mostly, did some on the elliptical machine and lifted weights a little. I really had no idea what I was doing, so I started reading books and articles on exercise and weight loss. This worked very well for a couple of months, but I quickly got tired of going there everyday and doing the same thing so I started walking some in the afternoons also.

Now remember, I didn't really enjoy getting hot, definitely not TWO times a day (health club in the morning, walking in the afternoon.) So, I started out doing what I thought might work. I knew I would NEVER continue to exercise for myself but I knew if I was doing it for the Lord, I just might. I would take my IPOD loaded with Christian music with me for these walks, and I would tell the Lord, "This is a sacrifice of praise to You. Your Word says to give myself as a holy sacrifice, so that is what I am doing". I would walk and l praise the Lord. One day I read in a magazine that jogging burns many more calories than walking so I thought, "I wonder if I could jog?" I started jogging. I would jog very little. I would count mailboxes, "I'm gonna jog to the third mailbox." As soon as I ran out of breath I would quit and get my breath, then start jogging again. It got to the point that I was able to actually jog a half a mile without stopping! I was soo proud of myself! What an accomplishment! This jogging thing became a bit of a personal challenge for me. It got to the point that I was so proud of what I was doing that I actually looked forward to going out and pushing myself a little more! I jogged five days a week, as much as I could stand. I remember when I made it a whole mile without stopping. WOW!! What a day! Of course, I thought I would die there on the concrete when I stopped running, but it felt so good! It was such an accomplishment! **The funny thing about exercise is it tricks your brain a little.** When you are exercising correctly and working out, you don't want to eat bad! You want to reward your body and nourish it for the hard work. That is why I exercise in the morning. To trick my mind into wanting to eat right all day long! I jogged that first mile without stopping, keep in mind I was still a plus size woman, a size 16W, but I was eating right and jogging and really feeling good about myself! WOW! Do you know what happens when you start feeling good about yourself? Your brain is tricked again! You want to keep taking good care of that self! You want to exercise it and eat healthy because you are proud of that self! Somewhere along the way my sacrifice of praise to the Lord became a JOY! I looked forward to that time. I still do.

There will be times you have a plateau. Just keep working through that. Often you need to add more "good" fat or just change up your routine a little to get things moving again. The one thing I want to tell you though is no matter what, do NOT give up!

I've talked to many people who tell me for medical reasons, or health issues that they can't run. Well, that's ok. Running wasn't the answer here. It was just the exercise that I chose to go with and what I really enjoy. You could walk, go for a swim, ride the bike, go to a gym. The key is to get moving. One thing to note is I had exercised many times in my life and not lost weight. At one point several years ago, I got so disgusted that I gave up. I was eating 1200 calories a day and walking 50 minutes on a treadmill five days a week.

One thing I learned through this journey is you have to trick your body and metabolism. I change my workout routine every 6 weeks or so. My body will get used to one thing and then I change it up. I must give my metabolism something to do, so it doesn't get bored and go to sleep! For the entire year that I lost the final 96 pounds I would eat 1300 calories on Tuesday and Thursday and 1500 on all other days. I did my heavy workouts (core ball training and weight lifting) on Monday, Wednesday and Friday. I knew I needed to eat a little more calories. On the weekends I wanted to enjoy my meals... when I started jogging more, I added more calories. I went to 1500 on those two days and 1700 on the other days.

The thing here is if your body feels like you are starving it, it will hold on to what you have. Eating 1200 calories a day was NOT enough and walking for 50 minutes a day, every day, was the same thing. My body got bored with that and quit losing weight. The popular topic of working out right now is interval training. We will talk more about that in the next chapter. One thing that will encourage you, is with time, people you haven't seen in a while won't even recognize you. I have passed many people in stores who look right at me, but don't know who I am until I speak to them. If you feel overwhelmed with information don't worry. I'm just telling you my story right now. I'm going to give you detailed lists and easy to follow plans at the end of the book to get you started.

CHAPTER THOUGHTS:

I will buy a cute journal or notebook to begin keeping track of all of my exercise and eating habits.

MAGIC TRICK NUMBER 5

-Interval Training

This is a HUGE Magic Trick! Your body burns more calories faster when you push it really hard for a few seconds then let it rest for a minute. There are many articles on-line about interval training. How many calories you should eat a day to lose weight and maintain your current weight. I will list some of these at the end of the book. Each person will have different numbers, so I couldn't list an answer here for everyone. If you will take the time to look at these websites you will get some ideas. Remember, the hardest part of exercise and moving at all is getting started. Once you get moving it feels so good you remember why you are doing it!

Here are a few websites about Interval Training that I found to be helpful. Also, listed below are a few sites that you can visit to help you figure out how much you should weigh, and how many calories you need to burn every day to lose weight or maintain your current weight.

This website will help you find out how many calories you should consume in a day: http://nutrition.about.com/library/bl_nutrition_guide.htm

This website will help you determine how many calories are burned for certain exercises: http://www.nutristrategy.com/activitylist4.htm

This website will further explain Interval Training: http://exercise. about.com/od/intervaltrainingworkouts/a/Interval- Training.htm

Website to determine your BMI (Body Mass Index):

http://www.nhlbisupport.com/bmi/

MAGIC TRICK NUMBER 6

-You Have Got To Talk To Yourself.

The tongue can bring death or life;... Proverbs 18:21a NLT
You are going to talk to yourself anyway, you just need to know the best things to say to yourself. Everyday, do you decide whether or not you are going to sleep that night? Do you wake up in the morning and think, "Hmmm, I wonder if I will feel like sleeping tonight? I wonder if I should?" Or do you ever think, "I don't want to fool with that. Sleep takes so much time. What a waste. It is not important. There are other things I should be doing." Isn't that ridiculous? But we will tell ourselves those things to get out of exercise.

To change your life you have to see exercise as being just as important as sleeping. There is no debate in your head if it is going to happen. You have to decide, today, that exercise is now a part of your life. I exercise five days a week. Many magazines and articles talk about taking two days off during the week. Many of them suggest that you not take the days of rest off together, but rather spread them out in the middle of the work-out week. Yes, this sounds like a great plan, but I know my chances of being 'too busy' on Saturday and Sunday (for me as a Worship Pastor) are too great for me to risk that. I always choose those days as rest days. There have been times because of meetings or travel that I have had to take off another day of the week, so I am sure to make up that day on Saturday. I work out or exercise five days a week. **Exercise must be as much of your**

routine as sleeping and brushing your teeth. No debate...just do it! I would tell myself while I was exercising especially on the days I didn't feel like it, "This is only 45 minutes of my day then I will feel sooo good that I did it" And that always worked. I can do anything for a limited amount of time.

NEVER say to yourself, "oh no, I've got to do this everyday for the rest of my life?" That can be scary for anyone. Just remind and tell yourself, "this is only 30 minutes of my day or 45 minutes of my day" - "I can do this!" ....I can do all things through Christ....

Another important thing to tell yourself, and I found myself telling other people, "I can eat whatever I want. There are no restrictions! I am NOT on a diet, I have just changed my habits and what I choose to eat!" I CAN eat that cupcake or that bowl of ice cream if I want it, I just don't want it!" You see, if you tell yourself all the time what you can't have you will be sad and feel deprived. If you remind yourself that you can have those things, you just don't want them everyday, then rather than feel deprived, you will feel empowered!! You have given yourself the power to say no and make a good choice!

CHAPTER THOUGHTS:

MAGIC TRICK NUMBER 7

Present Your Body As A Sacrifice.

S o whether you eat or drink, or whatever you do, do it all for the glory of God. 1 Corinthians 10:31 NLT

Changing your body is the best that you can give God! I plead with you to give your bodies to God because of all he has done for you. Let them be a living and holy sacrifice—the kind he will find acceptable. This is truly the way to worship him. Romans 12:1 NLT

You must be willing to present your body to God! Give Him your whole body! I would tell myself when I was exercising, "This is only 30 minutes of my day!" or, "This is only one hour of my day and Lord it is for you! It is worship to you. I am changing my body to please you. As a sacrifice of praise to You. It is my reasonable service. The least that I can do for you for all that you have done for me!"

A prayer to pray: Lord, today I present my body to You as a living sacrifice. Holy and pleasing to You. I appreciate all that You have done for me and all that You have given me, and this is the least that I can do for You. Today I give You my body, my heart, soul, mind, strength and energy to use for Your glory. Use all of me to bring honor and glory to Your name. Let my life be profitable for Your kingdom and let Your will be done in my life!

Someone very wise once said, "Knowledge is Power"....

Proverbs 19:2 Enthusiasm without knowledge is no good; haste makes mistakes. One of my best friends ordered a years subscription to Runners World for me. That was the best gift I have received in a long time. Reading that every month and having it sitting around to look at daily kept me focused and reminded me of what I was doing. Having a magazine laying around with a huge beautiful CAKE on the front cover worked against my goal. Remember, this is all about changing the old you into the new you.

What are some changes you can make? Stop and think about that for a minute. What are some simple changes that you can make that will help you reach your goals? Write them here.

_____

_____

_____

_____

_____

_____

I get online fairly regularly to look up 'healthy recipes'. One of my favorites has been veggie lasagna. Most every Tuesday evening I watch the Biggest Loser. I look at these people and see where they started and how far they have come. I memorize scripture or at least tape it to my mirrors and walls, so that I can be empowered by the Word of God. I hang quotes from other healthy people in my workout room at home.

Your goal should never again be, "to lose weight on this quick fix diet and then get back to life." No, that will not work. You must be wiling to attain knowledge to make permanent changes in your life and NEVER go back. It's not going to be a 'quick fix" but it will be a fix that can last a lifetime! I cannot even tell you how many times people have asked me, "are you still dieting or are you maintaining"?

I always say the same thing. "Neither. I changed my habits and my life. I'm just living my new life." My husband tells people, "She is basically an all out health nut." I'm not sure that is completely true, but I do consider everything I put into my mouth. I also consider what exercise I am doing daily and with every decision I ask myself, "Does this line up with my new goals to make and keep the new and improved me?"

Chapter Thoughts:

SOME EXPECTED CHANGES TO LOOK FOR

My husband is the greatest man on the earth. He has loved me from the beginning of our relationship. I was fat when we met and until a year and a half ago, was fat the previous 18 years of marriage. He never loved me less or acted any differently whether I lost 40 pounds or gained 50. He remained faithful, adoring, and loving towards me through it all, but I was unhappy with myself.

My husband and I had to have many discussions on what we could now do to 'connect'. All of our dating and married life we had connected over food. Dinners out, fun afternoon trips to the beach and Krispy Kreme, a trip to the ice cream store, a bowling date so we could eat the awesome hamburgers and Philly Beef Steak Sandwich! You see, our whole life revolved around food. We had to find ways to reconnect and find ways to go on dates that didn't involve fattening foods! During this transformation we had a few months of painful pruning and changing. We had to learn to connect in ways that didn't include food, and I had to learn to reassure my husband that just because I was changing did not mean I needed him any less. I knew we were having this struggle but couldn't figure out how to put words on his feelings or mine. I wasn't sure how to handle it because I knew I wasn't going back to the old me, but because I was still learning how to be the new me, I didn't have the answers we needed. So again, I prayed and asked the Lord what I should do and what was the best plan to handle this. Lucky for him (ha)

I am a huge fan of the Biggest Loser. Let me say that I basically despise reality television, but it is so inspiring to me to see these people and the transformations they make. I don't really like all the drama they include in the show to make it 'entertaining' but there really is a lot in there to learn from if you watch closely. On one of the episodes I was watching, around this time of a huge part of my weight loss, Jillian (the female trainer for the show) had gone home with one of the contestants to talk to his family. They were having the same issues! The wife felt that because her husband had changed so much that she felt she was left behind and wondered if he even needed her anymore. Jillian then began to tell how this happens all the time. In almost every case, that it was not an isolated instance. I was so happy to hear that. (Don't think the Lord can't answer your prayers through television and reading). Now I knew what to do. I spent days giving my husband undivided attention. Inviting him to walk with me and run with me. We even went skating one night (he LOVES skating and I hate it) but I wanted him to know that even though I had changed, he was still my number one man. That just because my body changed did not mean my heart for him had changed. That seemed to be the perfect solution, and we have not had a problem with that in many months. Even this afternoon we have a date planned to go bike riding on some nearby trails. I committed at that time to eat out with him once a week or so. I try to choose a restaurant that lists their nutritional values online and I look over the menu to see what is the best choice to eat, then know what I am going to order before I ever step foot in the restaurant.

Many of my relationships changed. I didn't have time to talk on the phone for a couple of hours everyday as I had previously done for years. The time I spent previously talking on the phone I was now exercising or making a menu for the week, or reading the Bible or an encouraging article. Many of my friends and family got upset with me and thought maybe I was trying to isolate myself. That wasn't the case, I just had to change my priorities. When I ask you are you ready for a change, I'm not just asking you that, it is something you must really consider! Stop making excuses. The time to change is now.

You have to be willing to make drastic changes! If you will commit to do it, you won't regret it! You will be so pleased with the changes you will never want to go back! The hardest, scariest step is the first one. The first one is making the decision to change. To never go back.

When I first started out I began using the "core" or "stability" ball. This is SUCH a fun, almost painless way to exercise, especially when you are first getting started. There was a deacon in our church that owned a glass company. He very graciously ordered, made, delivered, cut and hung custom mirrors for my workout area. I originally set up a corner in my bedroom for my work out area. You don't know me, but I have been pretty strict about how things look in my house. Up until this point I would have never allowed random mirrors on the wall and an area for exercise to invade my bedroom, but I was a changed woman. After the first year, I was so attached to working out, and it had become such a huge part of who I was, that I got rid of my kitchen table, moved our dining table to the kitchen area and changed the entire formal dining room into a work out room. We moved the mirrors to those walls, we added a treadmill, weight bench, free weights, the works! My family also now enjoys the room as well. So, my question for you, "Are you really ready to change?" "Are you ready to make permanent changes that might be difficult or uncomfortable in the beginning, but will ultimately lead to the new you, you have been dreaming of?"

I remember when I first started losing weight. As my clothes got too big, I would immediately get rid of them. I would give them to other people or put them in a consignment shop. That has been a great way to keep my running equipment purchased. About every 6 months, you will need new shoes and running bras, so in that time I have usually sold enough clothes to go get the money and purchase what I need. In the past years of losing and gaining, I have kept my clothes or at least the nicer stuff when I lost weight, "in case I need it again, in case I gain the weight back." Once I made up my mind to make the change, going back has no longer been an option. Once I lost the first 30 pounds, and had to get rid of basically my whole closet, that was very hard. I was so excited to not be able to wear any of my clothes anymore, but just as much as I was excited, I was scared. You see, once I got rid of an entire wardrobe I had to be prepared to never go back. There would be nothing to go back to! It took me a couple of weeks to get rid of the stuff. I kept it in bags in my closet. I can't explain why this was such a scary step, but it was. I did keep one pair of my favorite jeans that I wore all the time so I could hold them up in front of me to show how much weight I had lost! That is fun! After I got rid of that first set of clothes, it got easier every time. I started shopping at thrift stores because I didn't want to spend lots of money on clothes that I would only be wearing a short amount of time! I had friends and family who were so proud of me that they would buy me new clothes or just give me some of theirs to get me through to the next phase.

There have been so many spiritual changes as well. Wow, this is where the most fun changes for me have been. I start my day EVERYDAY, everyday with my best friend Jesus. I wake up early on busy days and sit in a 'prayer chair' that I have set up in a corner in our bedroom. I read the Bible and devotional books there. I pray, listen to inspiring music and just sit in His presence everyday. I KNOW that I can't make it on my own power and strength. I know that without Him I will fail! I will make bad choices. I will go in the wrong direction. There have been days that I have failed even after having been in His presence. So I am very aware of how much His guidance in my life means.

The difference I have now is when I do fail I don't heap guilt and condemnation on myself. For instance, when I'm walking through the mall, and the "Cookie Shop" is calling my name as I walk past it two times with good self control, but on that third time I have to have a cookie, when I do that, I just talk to myself. Remember, I told you earlier how you are going to talk to yourself in some way or the other. You have to choose to say good, helpful things to yourself. So now instead of saying,

"You loser! You failure! Do you have any idea how many calories are in that cookie that you just ate? Why did you do that? You are so stupid. You may as well eat five more and throw in the towel!" No, now I say, "Well, that cookie was good and I did enjoy it! Yum! It really hit the spot. Now, I'm going to walk this mall two more times, quickly, to burn off some of those calories that I just enjoyed!" So I walk and never think about it again.

Life was meant to be enjoyed!!

There was a mindset that I lived with for years. I always thought that people who were thin and healthy were just born that way. I thought that those people never had to work to keep themselves that way. I thought that either you were born with the healthy right body and you could eat whatever you wanted or you were born with a body like mine (at that time) and you could diet or eat bad, either way you were going to be fat. Basically I thought I was just born to be 'big'. I have learned through this experience that my thought process was all wrong. Once I lost the 100 pounds and got to the weight I wanted to reach, I don't have to worry as much with all of that. I do my exercise each day, and I keep my calories in check by eating healthy, natural foods with lots of fruits and vegetables. I have found however, that if I chose to have a day where I eat terribly, that I do not immediately gain 10 pounds. That I can enjoy treats and still remain at a healthy weight. Sometimes I don't feel as good in my body because once you remove sugar and chemicals from your body you realize how good you actually feel and it isn't until you put them back in that you realize how bad they make you feel. I guess what I'm trying to say is **you can change**. Just because you can't imagine how it can happen right now, and you know you have tried over and over in the past to no avail, it can happen.

You must take the time everyday to allow the Lord to change you. You don't have the power to do it yourself. If you did, you wouldn't be reading this, but HE does and if you are a Christian, you have His power inside of you, so through Him you can do this!! You can change! Are you willing to do what it takes? Are you willing to sit with Him everyday to let that happen? Are you willing to read His Word and do what it says?

CHAPTER THOUGHTS:

JUST BE FREE!

Christ has set us free to live a free life. So take your stand! Never again let anyone put a harness of slavery on you. Galatians 5:1 The Message

What is the literal definition of the word "Freedom?" It is exemption from obligation, unrestricted use. If you have given your life to Jesus Christ, asked Him to take over your whole life, change your mind and your way of thinking, then you are free from the obligation of being chained to over eat. According to Romans 6:1-14, you have the power to make the choice, the choice to walk away from sin and temptation. You have the power to overcome the temptation to eat unhealthy foods and to sit on the couch watching 2 hours of television rather than exercise. You have the power to choose to spend time with the Lord asking Him to change the way you think rather than be on facebook for an hour. You have been given the power to choose! You have the power!! Will you use it?

I have seen miracles. My son Andrew, who is now 11 years old was healed of cancer 10 years ago. The doctors at Sacred Heart Hospital in Pensacola, FL, told us to take him home and enjoy the last few months we were going to have with him because there was nothing more they could do. The Lord miraculously healed him. Totally! He is cancer free today and has been for many years. I have SEEN miracles!! Several people have been healed of cancer in our church, so I know God can do anything. Because I have faith and knowledge of what Christ can do, I prayed many times, "Lord, You can raise the dead! You raised Lazarus from the dead after four days! You healed blinded eyes, You opened deaf ears, You have done miracles that I can't even name! You healed my son from cancer!! You have healed other people! I KNOW you can heal me. Will you please help me? When I wake up tomorrow I would love for you to just take off 40 pounds. That would help me get started, and I will tell people that You did!! I will give You the glory! You said if I had faith I could move mountains, so I speak to this fat mountain!" I'm serious, I have prayed this and MORE than once or twice...many times! Boy, am I glad that the Lord didn't do that. He always knows what is best for us. I would have missed so much over the past couple of years. So much learning and knowledge of who Christ is. I would have missed much and I'm glad that He chose to heal me through a process of learning. A healing process of freedom.

Ephesians 4:22-24...throw off your old sinful nature and your former way of life, which is corrupted by lust and deception. [23] Instead, let the Spirit renew your thoughts and attitudes. [24] Put on your new nature, created to be like God—truly righteous and holy.

I am living proof that God can and WILL break destructive habits in your life. Destructive habits lead to sin and further separate you from Christ, thus making it virtually impossible to fulfill the destiny He has laid before you! You have to be willing to change what you can and be willing to throw off the old and take on the new!

If it is your hearts desire to lose weight, then read carefully these verses...

Psalm 37:4 NLT Take delight in the LORD, and he will give you your heart's desires.

Romans 12:2 Don't copy the behavior and customs of this world, but let God transform you into a new person by changing the way you think. Then you will learn to know God's will for you, which is good and pleasing and perfect.

This means that anyone who belongs to Christ has become a new person. The old life is gone; a new life has begun!

2 Corinthians 5:17 NLT

There are many scriptures for you to stand on and promises that the Lord WILL give you the power to change if you really want it. Another thing I have done is taken scriptures like these, and inserted my name so that I would be praying God's perfect will over my life. I typed these up and put them on my bathroom mirror, on the mirror in my room, on my computer screen at work, anywhere and everywhere that I would see them clearly. You see, God's Word will do the supernatural changing as you do the natural changing, making you into the new creature you want and desire to be! Here are some examples of these verses and how I applied them to my life. You can change them to apply to your life as well!

Pray this prayer today and begin telling yourself this everyday.

I choose today to throw off my old nature. My old nature would go to food to eat when I was upset. My old nature would rent a movie and go home to watch it to lose myself in the drama when I was upset. My old nature would turn to food for comfort, but I am choosing to throw off that nature. I choose to remove myself from that former way of life! It is corrupted by lust and deception. For it only causes me to continue to gain weight and stay in other forms of bondage. It does not give me the permanent freedom and comfort that I desire. So instead, I choose today to be renewed by the Spirit of God. Father, I ask You to renew my thoughts and my very attitude as I read your Word. Speak to me, let it change who I am, making me more like You. I put on my new nature today. I was created to be like God, in His image, truly righteous and holy.

Prayer from Psalm 37:4, Lord, today I will sit at Your feet before I do anything else with my day. I will delight in You. As I delight in You, make my heart like Yours and my desires Your desires so you can fulfill me!

Prayer from Romans 12:2, Thank You Father that I have been given power by Your Spirit to break free from copying what the world has to offer. I do not have to live with it's customs to eat fast food, fried food and be lazy, but I can be a new person. You are changing the way I think to be more like You, to live my life to please You and serve others. You want me to know Your will and I thank You for changing the way I think, so that I can know Your will for my life.

Prayer from 2 Corinthians 5:17, I belong to Christ, therefore I am a new creature! My old life, old habits, old way of thinking is gone! My new life begins today! I choose to let Christ lead me and speak to me everyday. I will obey what he says and continue to change my old, bad habits to make new ones!

Remember, it is a process. It took me many months to look in the mirror and not see the 'fat' Heather. Even a year later I would have the boys compare me to other women while we are out, "Do I look like her? Am I that size?" It takes a while to get used to the changes. Also, I thought that losing weight was going to bring me instant happiness. It didn't. However, God used this process to draw me closer to Him than ever before, and THAT has brought me true joy!

SECRET HINTS AND PRACTICAL TIPS

Carry a snack bag. Go buy a cute bag or ice chest. When my boys were little I NEVER left the house without a bag full of snacks for them. Treat yourself that way, pretend you are a toddler. You cannot leave the house unless you have a bag of snacks. Carry a pen and paper to track calories. Make it a cute little notepad so you will be excited to write down what you are eating.

Remember, the HUGE secret to weight loss is to eat less calories than you burn every day. So check out the website mentioned earlier to determine how many calories you should be eating and keep up with it. It will help you more than you know. You will be surprised how many calories you eat in a day if you don't track it carefully.

Reward yourself! Give yourself treats! I remember the first time that I ate a treat was at my grandfather's 80th birthday party. When I got home that night I felt like a failure! I had eaten cake, not just one piece either, many pieces. I thought for sure when I woke up my fairy tale would be over and I would be back to my original size overnight because I had that cake. Guess what? When I woke up, it was a new day. I hadn't even gained a pound! Now, if you have a 'treat' everyday that probably wouldn't be the case, but it is ok to reward yourself. If you have worked out all five days and stuck to your calorie goals for the week, don't be afraid to go have an ice cream cone! Don't be afraid to eat a candy bar. You will find as I did, that the things you think you want, won't taste the same. They lose their flavor and they are not as good as you remember and they make you sick! You get used to healthy things and not oil and butter, so when you add that to your diet it makes you feel a little queasy. I remember after that party where I ate a couple of pieces of cake, I had to eat Rolaids all night!

Just so I could sleep.

This brings me to the 'purging' story I mentioned earlier. We had a band concert at my son's school for Christmas. They served a dessert bar full of homemade desserts during the concert. I just want to say I felt like I had stepped onto the set of the Biggest Loser and was given a temptation challenge, and I must admit, I failed the challenge. I had one dessert and that was ok. The longer I sat there, I would take a bite of my son's dessert, then my husband's. They would go back for seconds and thirds and the stuff they were getting was so good. So I would go back too. I don't even know how many desserts I had that night but I know one thing, by the time I got home I was SICK. LITERALLY nauseas! I walked around the house a little trying to get comfortable. I couldn't. All that grease and sugar was just stuck, and wouldn't do down. I was remorseful. I knew I had given way to gluttony that night. I didn't have a treat, I ate like a HOG! I decided I was going to have to purge some of that so I could breath. (now you should know that I have never had the ability to be a bulimic because I HATE to vomit). When I was pregnant with my boys I vomited enough for a lifetime, and I would be fine if I never had to do it again! That night however, I was just sick and knew I needed relief. So I went to the bathroom trying to think of all the grossest stuff I had ever seen, bent over trying to vomit. Nothing. Even though that food was 'right there' it would NOT come up. So I stood back up and as I did I heard the Lord speak to me in an almost audible voice that He was going to use this to help me to learn not to do this again. That I was NOT going to vomit no matter how hard I tried and He was not going to take away the 'sick' feeling, it would have to just work it's way out. He was going to use this as a reminder of feeling the sickness for the next time I was presented with this situation. Well, first of all, I have no intentions of ever attending a 'dessert bar' again.

That is just as crazy as sending a former alcoholic to a free open bar for the night. I mean, there may be times you could handle that, but why even make yourself? Just avoid the temptation altogether. If the time ever comes that I am forced to attend a 'dessert bar' again I can assure you I will NOT forget the way I felt that night. So, my lesson was learned and the message I can present to you is enjoy your treat, just one at a time, or your treat will be a misery to you!

(Bulimia is a serious disease. This disease often kills people much faster than being overweight. If you do have a problem with Bulimia, talk to a trusted friend today. You can be free from this as well.)

When eating out, make it a game to find the healthiest meal on the menu. See what would be the best for you. I have really enjoyed this trick! I will go online and check out the nutrition guides for different restaurants in town and see what I can eat. If a particular place we are going does not have a menu or nutritional guide listed online, I will try to pick what I believe, from my learned knowledge, the healthiest meal would be.

If you are like me, sometimes all of this information can be overwhelming and still leave you wondering where to start. I am a 'list' person. I like to see my goals and accomplish them task by task. So, I have compiled a list of all of the things I have talked about in this book to make it easier for you. The most important thing to remember, is you are not making changes in a hurry. You are not making temporary adjustments. You are making permanent life changing decisions so don't be in a rush to get through these steps. You have your whole life ahead of you to make the changes. The List:

1. Pray and fast. Remember I talked about how important prayer and fasting is. You need time to allow the 'bad' stuff to get out

of your system and allow your taste buds to crave healthy things. Pray and ask the Lord to give you a plan that will work for you during this time. Be willing to stick with the fast as long as possible. Do not starve yourself or go on a complete fast during this time. This is simply to begin teaching you self control and to kill your flesh, not to starve yourself. A Daniel fast will do that and will keep you healthy for an extended period of time. (if you are diabetic you may need to make a few adjustments to reduce the carb intake). See your physician if you are unclear based on your medical needs.

2. Spend time with the Lord allowing Him to change your thinking and your habits. Everyday you need to have time where you are alone with God, praying, reading His Word, asking Him to change you. Get a devotional book, some Christian music and your Bible. Or, you can start out like I did. I would read my Bible for a few minutes, then head outside for my sacrifice of worship in the form of walking, then later running. Don't allow your flesh to tell you, you don't have time to spend with the Lord. You do. Cut out one sit-com, facebook time, one phone call a day, one novel reading session. Ask the Lord what is an area that you can eliminate in your life to give you more time to devote to Him. I PROMISE He will reveal it to you. He LOVES to spend time with you and is just waiting on you to come be with Him. He wants to help you reach your goals and dreams. You have to be willing to let Him. If you want to change who you are you have to change your habits. As you are spending time with the Lord everyday, ask the Lord to reveal where you allowed these chains to first be latched on to you. Spend quiet time in His presence and let Him give you the answers. When He gives them to you, write it down or type it out. Find a Godly friend that you trust to talk to and have them pray with you and offer insight. These places may be very scary, so be prepared to let the Lord hold your hand

and bring you healing. Again, He wants to. He loves you and wants to heal you. Once you discover where these chains and this bondage to food came from, forgive. Forgive the person or the people. Forgive yourself. Put the past in the past. Discover it, face it, kill it, then bury it forever and move forward. If you have never been successful in the past making changes for yourself, start out doing it as an act of worship for Him. He deserves our best, and when you give Him your best, He will honor it and help you!

3. Develop an eating plan that will last a life time. Don't set out to only eat 1000 or 1200 calories a day. Make realistic goals. You can't live off that few calories everyday of your life, so don't try to do it now. You are not on a temporary diet, you are making permanent changes. Hold yourself accountable. I keep cute little notepads in my kitchen. In the beginning I wrote down how many calories, fat grams, protein grams, fiber and carbs were in EVERYTHING I put in my mouth. Now that I have gotten to my goal weight I only keep up with the calories. I learned so much writing all of that down that I don't need to write it all now. I pretty much KNOW what is in the foods I eat, but I keep those cute little notepads to keep track of what I eat. If I decide to have a cupcake at a birthday party, I write that down. I want to remember I ate that in case a cookie starts calling my name later. I can see where I have already had a treat for that day, and I am much more likely to say no the second time around if I see on my note pad: Banana 70 calories, yogurt, 100 calories, cupcake 350 calories. See? When you see it written down it makes that yummy cupcake not look so delicious!

4. Get moving. Move. Exercise. Again, don't allow your mind to wake up and have a debate on whether or not you are going to. Just do it. Make it as much as a part of your day as sleeping and brushing your teeth. You will do it no matter what. Don't get stuck with what exercise you will do, just do something. If

nothing else go walk. Find a place with a few hills. Remember what I told you about interval training? If you can't find a place with hills, then count out mailboxes where you will speed walk and get your heart rate up for 30 seconds at a time, then bring it back down. Repeat that throughout a 30 minute interval in the beginning. Don't worry about what you will do when 30 minutes isn't enough anymore, TRUST me, when that time comes you will be WANTING to exercise!!

5. Don't give up. Don't quit. Did you eat 3,000 calories today because you had a bad day? Did you go on vacation and blow it? Well, feel bad for 2 minutes, then get back on your routine tomorrow. Remember, you are not in a race to lose weight. This is not a 'lose 80 pounds in 5 days' competition. It's a lifetime of changes. One bad day is not going to hurt you, what will devastate your plan is to have one bad day and decide to give up, making it two bad days, then three, on and on. Don't quit!! YOU CAN DO THIS!!!!

6. Surround yourself with people who are proud of you! People who tell you they are proud. Be prepared that some people that you thought would be supportive may begin to feel threatened by the changes they see in you!

    My husband always says, "People hate other's success. Don't take it personal. It wasn't meant to hurt you, they are just trying to make themselves feel better." Take their hatefulness as a compliment. So true! Just smile and keep going.

7. Talk to yourself. Tell yourself you can do it. Don't talk like an overweight person in chains. Talk like the skinny, healthy, free person you dream of being. What you believe in your heart is what you are and what you will become. I have literally told myself out loud in my kitchen, "Heather! You do NOT want that pre-packaged, boxed dessert! You don't even like those! Put it down and get an orange. You are just bored." Literally, it works!!

I tell myself almost on a daily basis during my running that I can make it. I tell myself things like, "Once you get on top of this hill you get to go down. You remember how easy it is to go down? You can breath again then, you are almost there." Tell yourself the things you need to hear! If you blow it, tell yourself, "It's okay, tomorrow you have got to get back on track, and you are running (or walking) an extra lap for those wasted calories." (can you tell I've used that one before?)

FOREVER FREEDOM....IT'S YOUR CHOICE!

You have to choose to stay free. You see, you can be in prison, serve your time for a crime, then be released. At that moment an ex-prisoner is free! They will not have to go back to prison for that crime ever again. However, if they commit the crime again, and are caught, they will have to serve more time.

Once the Lord sets you free, you are free. You never have to go back to those prison chains again. It is up to you to remain free. You see, for instance, if someone robs a bank because they felt like they needed some money and fast, they can serve their time in the prison for that crime and after a few years be released. At that time, they can choose to be free forever and NEVER even consider robbing a bank again, or, they can begin to think, "Boy, if I had of changed only this or that I might not have gotten caught. I really need some money again, I wonder if there is a way I could rob another bank and get some money." You see, their thoughts have now led them right back to the same road to lead them back to prison. In the same way, the Lord sets us free. You can be free, but you can also choose to begin to think destructive thoughts, plan destructive plans and live in destructive habits that will lead you right back to your prison. I have heard many people in the past say, "The Lord did not grant me freedom. I must not be good enough. He must not be real." I have heard many statements like those. The Lord ALWAYS grants freedom. Unfortunately, the choice to remain free can sometimes be very difficult and we put ourselves right back down the road to prison cells. Then we blame the only One who can truly set us free.

What would happen if that same ex-prisoner said, "Oh thank the Lord I learned my lesson and I NEVER want to go back to prison. I will work three jobs and earn the money I need before I will even consider thinking of robbing a bank again," and then they do not return to that thought? Nothing! They are still free!

You have the choice. The Lord grants you freedom. Will you receive it? Do you want it?

So if the Son sets you free, you are truly free.... John 8:36 NLT

SPECIAL THANKS...

I would like to say thank you to my Freedom Giver, Jesus Christ! This accomplishment was only possible because of Him! I give Him all glory! I will do my best to spread His freedom message as long as I live. I will do my best to never again take His freedom for granted.

A very special thank you goes to my husband, Brian. He has loved me through every stage of life so far. He is always patient, kind and considerate of my feelings. He truly loves me as Christ loves the church. I have never doubted his love for me no matter how I felt about myself. He has always treated me as if I were the most beautiful, sexy woman on earth, even if I didn't believe it myself. It is because of his confidence and belief in me that I was able to find freedom! I have the greatest, most loving, caring husband in the world, and I know it! (I REALLY appreciate you editing for me at the last minute, even though you had a migraine...that is true love!) Thank you...I love you with all of my heart!

I would like to thank my sons, Aaron and Andrew, for loving me no matter what weight I have been. They have been so patient with me through all of the emotional turmoil, the grumpy days where I just wanted chocolate but couldn't have it. ☺ I love my three men/young men, more than anything in this world. I am blessed beyond all measure to have them in my life.

I would like to say thank you to my other family members and friends who have encouraged me over the past three years. Even though many of you have been around for years and have been a part of the yo-yo dieting events, you never reminded me of past failures. You just kept encouraging me to make it to the finish line. Thank you, to Dale and Paulette who gave me money to buy clothes throughout the journey. Thank you Sarah for purchasing my 123 FIT membership and giving me the jump start that I needed. Thank you for the wardrobes of clothes that you gave me as my closet no longer fit! Thank you Karen for listening and giving me a safe place to think out loud, for all of the prayers, guidance, godly wisdom, and supernatural encouragement to not give up, right when I needed it. I am pretty sure I would not have made it without you. I want to thank my dad and mom. I tell the Lord "thank you" on a regular basis for giving me Godly parents who loved me.

I would like to thank Bohannon Glass, Cantonment, FL, for donating wall sized mirrors, and installing them, for my work out space!